Twenty-Two Complete Session Scripts for Hypnotists

Joseph E. Sapp, JD CCH-AP

Copyright 2023, Joseph E. Sapp
ISBN 9798852940803

Table of Contents

FORWARD..13

INTRODUCTION..14

An Introduction to Hypnosis: Unveiling the Mystery and Power of the Mind......................16

The Art of Scripting in Hypnotherapy: Maximizing Effectiveness and Client Outcomes..19

Complete Session Scripts............................23

    ANXIETY SESSION 1................................24
    Pre-talk..24
    Induction...24
    Deepener..25
    Metaphors..26
    Direct Suggestions..................................26
    Indirect Suggestions...............................27
    Embedded Commands..........................27
    Post Hypnotic Suggestions......................27

- Awakener...27
- **ANXIETY SESSION 2**......................................29
  - Pre-talk...29
  - Induction...29
  - Deepener..30
  - Metaphors...30
  - Direct Suggestions....................................31
  - Indirect Suggestions..................................31
  - Embedded Commands.....................................31
  - Post Hypnotic Suggestions.............................32
  - Awakener..32
- **GRIEF SESSION 1**..34
  - Pre-talk...34
  - Induction...34
  - Deepener..35
  - Metaphors...36
  - Direct Suggestions....................................36
  - Indirect Suggestions..................................37
  - Embedded Commands.....................................37
  - Post Hypnotic Suggestions.............................37
  - Awakener..37
- **GRIEF SESSION 2**..39
  - Pre-talk...39
  - Induction...39
  - Deepener..40
  - Metaphors...40

   Direct Suggestions..................................41
   Indirect Suggestions.............................41
   Embedded Commands........................41
   Post Hypnotic Suggestions...................42
   Awakener..42
RELEASE TRAUMA SESSION 1....................44
   Pre-talk..44
   Induction...44
   Deepener...45
   Metaphors..46
   Direct Suggestions..................................46
   Indirect Suggestions.............................47
   Embedded Commands........................47
   Post Hypnotic Suggestions...................47
   Awakener..47
RELEASE TRAUMA 2.....................................49
   Pre-talk..49
   Induction...49
   Deepener...50
   Metaphors..50
   Direct Suggestions..................................51
   Indirect Suggestions.............................51
   Embedded Commands........................51
   Post Hypnotic Suggestions...................52
   Awakener..52
OVERCOMING ADDICTIONS 1.......................54

- Pre-talk..54
- Induction..54
- Deepener..55
- Metaphors..56
- Direct Suggestions...............................56
- Indirect Suggestions............................57
- Embedded Commands........................57
- Post Hypnotic Suggestions..................57
- Awakener..57

Overcoming Addiction 2.............................59

- Pre-talk..59
- Induction..59
- Deepener..60
- Metaphors..60
- Direct Suggestions...............................61
- Indirect Suggestions............................61
- Embedded Commands........................61
- Post Hypnotic Suggestions..................62
- Awakener..62

ATTRACTING ABUNDANCE 1.......................64

- Pre-talk..64
- Induction..64
- Deepener..65
- Metaphors..65
- Direct Suggestions...............................66
- Indirect Suggestions............................66

- Embedded Commands..................67
- Post Hypnotic Suggestions.......67
- Awakener.................................67

ATTRACT ABUNDANCE 2..........69

- Pre-talk...................................69
- Induction................................69
- Deepener................................70
- Metaphors...............................70
- Direct Suggestions..................71
- Indirect Suggestions...............71
- Embedded Commands..............72
- Post Hypnotic Suggestions.......72
- Awakener.................................72

CONFIDENCE BUILDING EGO STRENGTHENING 1..........74

- Pre-talk...................................74
- Induction................................74
- Deepener................................75
- Metaphors...............................75
- Direct Suggestions..................76
- Indirect Suggestions...............76
- Embedded Commands..............77
- Post Hypnotic Suggestions.......77
- Awakener.................................77

CONFIDENCE BUILDING EGO STRENGTHENING 2..........79

    Pre-talk..79
    Induction...79
    Deepener...80
    Metaphors..80
    Direct Suggestions..................................81
    Indirect Suggestions...............................81
    Embedded Commands............................82
    Post Hypnotic Suggestions......................82
    Awakener..82
RELEASING ANGER 1...................................84
    Pre-talk..84
    Induction...84
    Deepener...85
    Metaphors..85
    Direct Suggestions..................................86
    Indirect Suggestions...............................86
    Embedded Commands............................86
    Post Hypnotic Suggestions......................87
    Awakener..87
RELEASING ANGER 2...................................89
    Pre-talk..89
    Induction...89
    Deepener...90
    Metaphors..90
    Direct Suggestions..................................91
    Indirect Suggestions...............................91

- Embedded Commands..................91
- Post Hypnotic Suggestions......................92
- Awakener..................92

OVERCOMING ADVERSITY 1.......................94
- Pre-talk..................94
- Induction..................94
- Deepener..................95
- Metaphors..................95
- Direct Suggestions..................96
- Indirect Suggestions..................96
- Embedded Commands..................96
- Post Hypnotic Suggestions......................97
- Awakener..................97

OVERCOMING ADVERSITY 2.......................99
- Pre-talk..................99
- Induction..................99
- Deepener..................100
- Metaphors..................100
- Direct Suggestions..................101
- Indirect Suggestions..................101
- Embedded Commands..................101
- Post Hypnotic Suggestions......................102
- Awakener..................102

FINDING INSPIRATION 1...........................104
- Pre-talk..................104
- Induction..................104

- Deepener..105
- Metaphors..105
- Direct Suggestions..................................106
- Indirect Suggestions..............................106
- Embedded Commands.........................107
- Post Hypnotic Suggestions....................107
- Awakener...107

FINDING INSPIRATION 2..........................109

- Pre-talk..109
- Induction..109
- Deepener...110
- Metaphors..110
- Direct Suggestions................................111
- Indirect Suggestions..............................111
- Embedded Commands..........................112
- Post Hypnotic Suggestions....................112
- Awakener...112

THIRD EYE 1..114

- Pre-talk..114
- Induction..114
- Deepener...115
- Metaphors..115
- Direct Suggestions................................116
- Indirect Suggestions..............................116
- Embedded Commands..........................117
- Post Hypnotic Suggestions....................117

    Awakener..117
THIRD EYE 2..119
    Pre-talk..119
    Induction...119
    Deepener..120
    Metaphors..120
    Direct Suggestions................................121
    Indirect Suggestions.............................121
    Embedded Commands...........................122
    Post Hypnotic Suggestions...................122
    Awakener..122
RELAXATION 1......................................124
    Pre-talk..124
    Induction...124
    Deepener..125
    Metaphors..125
    Direct Suggestions................................126
    Indirect Suggestions.............................126
    Embedded Commands...........................126
    Post Hypnotic Suggestions...................126
    Awakener..127
RELAXATION 2......................................129
    Pre-talk..129
    Induction...129
    Deepener..130
    Metaphors..130

- Direct Suggestions...................................131
- Indirect Suggestions..............................131
- Embedded Commands...........................131
- Post Hypnotic Suggestions....................132
- Awakener...132
- **ABOUT THE AUTHOR**............................134
- **EDUCATION**...137

FORWARD

In today's fast-paced and increasingly complex world, people are faced with a myriad of challenges that can impact their emotional and psychological well-being. From managing stress and anxiety to overcoming grief and trauma, individuals are seeking effective and accessible tools to help them navigate life's ups and downs. As a result, there is a growing demand for skilled professionals who can provide guidance and support in addressing these issues.

Hypnosis has long been recognized as a powerful tool for personal transformation and healing. The practice of hypnosis taps into the subconscious mind, enabling individuals to access their inner resources and create lasting change in their lives. With the right guidance and support, hypnosis can provide a pathway to overcoming adversity and achieving personal growth.

"_More Hypnoscripts: Twenty-Two Complete Session Scripts for Hypnotists_" is a valuable resource for both experienced and aspiring hypnotists, providing a comprehensive collection of hypnosis session scripts designed to address a wide range of issues. This book offers a practical and effective approach to helping clients achieve their goals and overcome life's challenges.

INTRODUCTION

"*More Hypnoscripts: Twenty-Two Complete Session Scripts for Hypnotists*" is a unique and comprehensive guide that offers hypnotists a wealth of resources to enhance their practice and support their clients. This book contains 22 full session hypnosis scripts, each tailored to address a specific issue, such as anger management, overcoming grief, relaxation, stress relief, anxiety relief, confidence building, overcoming trauma, and overcoming adversity, among others.

Each script has been carefully crafted to ensure maximum effectiveness, drawing on the latest research and best practices in the field of hypnosis. The scripts are designed to be adaptable to individual clients' needs, allowing hypnotists to customize their approach and provide personalized support.

In addition to the session scripts, this book also includes an introduction to hypnosis and guidance on how to use the scripts effectively. This information is designed to support both experienced hypnotists and those new to the field, providing valuable insights and tips on how to create a successful and transformative hypnosis experience for clients.

"*More Hypnoscripts: Twenty-Two Complete Session Scripts for Hypnotists*" is an essential resource for anyone looking to expand their knowledge of hypnosis and enhance their ability to help clients overcome life's challenges. Whether you are a seasoned hypnotist or just starting your journey in this fascinating field, this book offers a wealth of practical tools and techniques that can help you make a real difference in the lives of those you serve.

An Introduction to Hypnosis: Unveiling the Mystery and Power of the Mind

Hypnosis, a widely misunderstood yet fascinating subject, has piqued the curiosity of many, often evoking images of stage performers and mind control. However, the reality of hypnosis is far from these misconceptions. As a natural state of focused attention and deep relaxation, hypnosis has a rich history and scientific basis, offering individuals a powerful tool for personal transformation and healing. This essay will provide an introduction to hypnosis, exploring its definition, history, science, and techniques.

To understand hypnosis, it is crucial to dispel the myths and misconceptions surrounding it. Hypnosis is neither mind control nor a loss of consciousness. Contrary to popular belief, clients cannot be forced to do something against their will or moral beliefs during hypnosis. In reality, hypnosis is a natural state of heightened focus and relaxation, similar to meditation or daydreaming. The hypnotic process relies on a client's suggestibility and imagination, allowing them to access their subconscious mind and create lasting change.

The history of hypnosis dates back to ancient civilizations, where early forms of hypnotic practices were used in Egypt and Greece. In the 18th century, Franz Anton Mesmer developed the concept of mesmerism, which laid the groundwork for modern hypnosis. James Braid, a Scottish surgeon, later coined the term "hypnosis" and developed the concept of suggestion in the 19th century. Over the years, prominent figures such as Sigmund Freud and Milton Erickson have contributed significantly to the field, shaping the practice of hypnosis as we know it today.

The science of hypnosis has also evolved over time, with ongoing research shedding light on its mechanisms and effectiveness. Hypnosis is believed to alter the brain's activity, inducing a state known as the hypnotic trance. This state affects perception, memory, and cognition, allowing clients to access and influence their subconscious mind. Numerous studies have demonstrated the efficacy of hypnosis for various issues and conditions, such as pain management, habit change, and mental health disorders. However, more research is needed to fully understand the complexities of hypnosis and its potential applications.

Hypnosis techniques are diverse, encompassing induction, deepening, and suggestion. Induction techniques guide clients into a state of deep relaxation and focused attention, while deepening techniques help clients achieve a deeper state of hypnosis. Suggestions, both direct and indirect, are used to influence clients' thoughts, feelings, and behaviors in a positive and empowering manner. The hypnotist plays a crucial role in guiding clients through the process, establishing rapport and trust, and adapting the session to meet their needs and goals.

Ethics and professionalism are paramount in the practice of hypnosis. Hypnotists must adhere to ethical guidelines and best practices, including informed consent, confidentiality, and respecting clients' boundaries. Ongoing professional development and staying current with advances in the field are essential to ensure the highest quality of care. Hypnotists must also recognize the limits of their expertise, making appropriate referrals when necessary and prioritizing client safety above all else.

In conclusion, hypnosis is a powerful and versatile tool for personal growth and healing. Far from the misconceptions of mind control and stage antics, hypnosis taps into the subconscious mind, enabling individuals to access their inner resources and overcome life's challenges. With a rich history and a growing body of scientific evidence supporting its effectiveness, hypnosis offers a valuable pathway for individuals seeking to transform their lives. As our understanding of hypnosis continues to deepen, so too does the potential to harness its power for the betterment of humankind.

The Art of Scripting in Hypnotherapy: Maximizing Effectiveness and Client Outcomes

Hypnotherapy, a powerful therapeutic approach that utilizes the power of hypnosis, has gained widespread recognition for its ability to facilitate personal growth and healing. At the heart of hypnotherapy lies the use of scripts, carefully crafted verbal guidance that helps clients access their subconscious mind and create lasting change. The proper use of scripts is vital to the success of a hypnotherapy session, requiring skillful adaptation, customization, and delivery. This essay will explore the importance of scripts in hypnotherapy, offering insights into their effective use for optimal client outcomes.

Preparing for a hypnotherapy session is the first step in ensuring the effectiveness of scripts. The therapist must create a comfortable and safe environment for the client, fostering a sense of trust and rapport. This foundation enables clients to feel at ease, increasing their receptivity to the therapist's guidance. Assessing the client's needs and goals is also essential, providing the therapist with valuable information to tailor the script accordingly.

Customizing scripts to suit individual clients and their specific issues is crucial in maximizing their impact. By incorporating client-specific language and imagery, therapists can enhance the effectiveness of the scripts, making them more personally relevant and meaningful. This level of customization requires the therapist to be attentive to the client's unique experiences, preferences, and communication style, adapting the script to resonate deeply with the client's subconscious mind.

The proper use of induction techniques is another key aspect of scripting in hypnotherapy. Induction techniques guide clients into a state of deep relaxation and focused attention, setting the stage for the therapeutic work to follow. Therapists must choose the most appropriate induction technique for each client, taking into account their level of suggestibility, comfort, and prior experience with hypnosis. By skillfully guiding clients into a hypnotic state, therapists can optimize the effectiveness of the scripts that follow.

Deepening techniques are an essential component of scripting in hypnotherapy, helping clients achieve a deeper state of hypnosis. The therapist must monitor and gauge the depth of the client's hypnotic state, adjusting the deepening techniques as needed to ensure the client remains receptive to the therapeutic suggestions. This level of attentiveness and adaptability is vital in maximizing the impact of the scripts and facilitating meaningful change.

Delivering suggestions and metaphors effectively is a critical aspect of scripting in hypnotherapy. The therapist must use clear, positive, and empowering language, ensuring that the suggestions align with the client's goals and values. Metaphors, stories, and analogies can be particularly powerful in hypnotherapy, tapping into the client's imagination and subconscious mind to create lasting change. The skillful delivery of suggestions and metaphors can make the difference between a successful hypnotherapy session and one that falls short of its intended outcomes.

Post-hypnotic suggestions and awakeners are the final components of effective scripting in hypnotherapy. Post-hypnotic suggestions are designed to reinforce the changes made during the session, helping clients integrate their new insights and behaviors into their daily lives. Awakeners, on the other hand, gently guide clients out of hypnosis and back to full awareness, ensuring a smooth transition and a positive conclusion to the session.

In conclusion, the proper use of scripts in hypnotherapy is vital to the success of the therapeutic process. By skillfully adapting, customizing, and delivering scripts, therapists can maximize their effectiveness and facilitate meaningful change for their clients. The art of scripting in hypnotherapy is a delicate balance of attentiveness, adaptability, and skill, requiring therapists to continually hone their craft and remain committed to their clients' well-being. As the field of hypnotherapy continues to evolve, so too will our understanding of the power of scripting and its potential to transform lives.

Complete Scripts Session

What follows are 22 complete session scripts as set out in the contents. There are two essential variations of each script presented. Customize and modify according to need.

ANXIETY SESSION 1

Pre-talk

Hello and welcome to this hypnosis session designed to help you reduce anxiety and feel more relaxed in your daily life. Before we begin, I want to ensure that you are in a comfortable and safe environment, free from any distractions. Make sure you are seated or lying down in a relaxed position. Remember, hypnosis is a natural state of relaxation and focus, and you are always in control. This session is about guiding you to discover your own inner resources for dealing with anxiety.

Induction

Now, let's begin. Close your eyes and take a few deep breaths. Inhale through your nose, and exhale through your mouth. With each breath, feel your body becoming more and more relaxed. Allow any tension or stress to simply melt away as you focus on your breathing.

As you continue to breathe, I'd like you to imagine a warm, soothing light at the top of your head. This light represents relaxation and comfort. As this light begins to spread, feel the muscles in your forehead and face relax. Allow this warm light to continue spreading down to your neck and shoulders, releasing any tension that may be stored there.

Deepener

The soothing light continues to move down your arms, through your chest and stomach, and into your hips and legs. With each breath, this warm light is filling your body, leaving you completely relaxed and at ease.

Now, imagine yourself at the top of a staircase with ten steps. Each step represents a deeper level of relaxation. As I count down from ten to one, you will descend the staircase, feeling more and more relaxed with each step.

10 - Taking the first step, feeling more relaxed.
9 - Deeper and deeper.
8 - Feeling lighter and more at ease.
7 - Your body and mind are becoming one.
6 - Halfway there, feeling completely relaxed.
5 - Deeper still, as you continue to descend.
4 - Almost at the bottom, feeling so peaceful.
3 - Just a few more steps.
2 - At the edge of complete relaxation.

1 - You have reached the bottom, feeling completely relaxed and at ease.

Metaphors

Imagine yourself in a beautiful garden, filled with vibrant colors and the soothing sounds of nature. This garden represents your mind, and each flower represents a positive thought or experience. As you wander through the garden, you notice that there are some weeds growing among the flowers. These weeds represent your anxiety and stress.

You have the power to remove these weeds, allowing your garden to flourish with positivity. As you pluck each weed from the ground, you feel a sense of relief and calmness wash over you. With each weed removed, your garden becomes more beautiful and serene, just like your mind.

Direct Suggestions

As you continue to relax, I want you to know that you have the ability to manage your anxiety. Each day, you are becoming more and more skilled at handling stress and maintaining a sense of calm. You are able to recognize when anxiety begins to surface and can take control before it overwhelms you.

Indirect Suggestions

You might find yourself discovering new ways to cope with anxiety, such as deep breathing, meditation, or physical activity. It's interesting how the mind can adapt and learn new techniques to maintain a sense of balance and calm.

Embedded Commands

You can feel confident in your ability to manage anxiety and stress. Trust your inner strength to guide you through difficult situations and remember that you are in control.

Post Hypnotic Suggestions

From this moment forward, whenever you feel anxiety beginning to surface, simply take a deep breath and remind yourself of your inner strength and ability to manage stress. You have the tools and resources to maintain a sense of calm and balance in your life.

Awakener

Now, it's time to return to full awareness. I will count from one to five, and with each number, you will become more and more awake, bringing with you the positive suggestions and feelings of relaxation.

1 - Beginning to awaken, feeling refreshed.
2 - Becoming more and more alert.
3 - Feeling your body and mind re-energize.
4 - Almost completely awake, feeling wonderful.
5 - Fully awake and alert, feeling refreshed and ready to face the day with a sense of calm and confidence.

Take a moment to stretch and enjoy the feeling of relaxation and rejuvenation. Remember, you have the power to manage anxiety and maintain a sense of balance in your life.

ANXIETY SESSION 2

Pre-talk

Welcome to this hypnosis session designed to help you reduce stress and find a sense of calm and balance in your life. Before we begin, ensure that you are in a comfortable, quiet space where you can fully relax without any interruptions. Remember, hypnosis is a natural state of focused relaxation, and you are always in control throughout the process. This session aims to guide you in tapping into your own inner resources to effectively manage stress.

Induction

Let's begin by finding a comfortable position, either sitting or lying down. Close your eyes and take a few slow, deep breaths. Inhale through your nose, and exhale through your mouth. With each breath, feel your body becoming more and more relaxed, allowing any tension or stress to simply dissipate.

As you continue to breathe, imagine a calming wave of relaxation gently washing over your body, starting at your head and gradually moving down to your toes. Feel this wave soothing every muscle, releasing any tension as it passes through.

Deepener

Now, picture yourself standing in front of a peaceful, calm lake. The water is so still that it perfectly reflects the sky above. This lake represents your mind, and the stillness of the water represents your inner calm.

Imagine picking up a small pebble and gently tossing it into the lake. As the pebble breaks the surface, ripples begin to form, spreading outwards. These ripples represent your stress and tension. However, just as the ripples gradually fade away, so too does your stress, leaving the water calm and still once again.

Metaphors

As you stand beside this peaceful lake, you notice a beautiful, strong tree nearby. This tree represents your inner strength and resilience. Just as the tree's roots anchor it firmly into the ground, your inner strength keeps you grounded and stable, even during times of stress.

The tree's branches stretch out towards the sky, symbolizing your ability to reach for new opportunities and experiences. As you observe the tree, you realize that it has weathered many storms, yet it continues to stand tall and strong. This is a reminder that you, too, can withstand life's challenges and emerge stronger and more resilient.

Direct Suggestions

As you continue to relax, know that you possess the ability to manage stress effectively. Each day, you are becoming more skilled at recognizing and addressing stressors in your life. You have the power to maintain a sense of balance and calm, no matter what challenges you may face.

Indirect Suggestions

It's fascinating how the mind can develop new strategies for coping with stress, such as engaging in relaxation techniques, practicing mindfulness, or seeking support from friends and loved ones.

Embedded Commands

Trust in your inner strength and resilience to help you navigate through stressful situations.

Remember that you have the power to create a sense of balance and calm in your life.

Post Hypnotic Suggestions

From now on, whenever you feel stress beginning to build, take a moment to pause and remind yourself of your inner strength and resilience. You have the tools and resources necessary to effectively manage stress and maintain a sense of balance in your life.

Awakener

It's time to return to full awareness. I will count from one to five, and with each number, you will become more and more awake, bringing with you the positive suggestions and feelings of relaxation.

1 - Beginning to awaken, feeling rejuvenated.
2 - Becoming more alert and aware.
3 - Feeling your body and mind re-energize.
4 - Almost completely awake, feeling refreshed and revitalized.
5 - Fully awake and alert, ready to face the day with a renewed sense of calm and balance.

Take a moment to stretch and enjoy the feeling of relaxation and rejuvenation. Remember, you

possess the power to manage stress and maintain a sense of balance in your life.

GRIEF SESSION 1

Pre-talk

Welcome to this hypnosis session designed to help you overcome grief and find healing. Before we begin, please ensure that you are in a comfortable and safe environment, free from any distractions. Make sure you are seated or lying down in a relaxed position. Remember, hypnosis is a natural state of relaxation and focus, and you are always in control. This session is about guiding you to discover your own inner resources for healing and moving forward.

Induction

Now, let's begin. Close your eyes and take a few deep breaths. Inhale through your nose, and exhale through your mouth. With each breath, feel your body becoming more and more relaxed. Allow any tension or stress to simply melt away as you focus on your breathing.

As you continue to breathe, I'd like you to imagine a warm, soothing light at the top of your head. This light represents relaxation and comfort. As this light begins to spread, feel the muscles in your forehead and face relax. Allow this warm light to continue spreading down to your neck and shoulders, releasing any tension that may be stored there.

Deepener

The soothing light continues to move down your arms, through your chest and stomach, and into your hips and legs. With each breath, this warm light is filling your body, leaving you completely relaxed and at ease.

Now, imagine yourself at the top of a staircase with ten steps. Each step represents a deeper level of relaxation. As I count down from ten to one, you will descend the staircase, feeling more and more relaxed with each step.

10 - Taking the first step, feeling more relaxed.
9 - Deeper and deeper.
8 - Feeling lighter and more at ease.
7 - Your body and mind are becoming one.
6 - Halfway there, feeling completely relaxed.
5 - Deeper still, as you continue to descend.
4 - Almost at the bottom, feeling so peaceful.
3 - Just a few more steps.
2 - At the edge of complete relaxation.

1 - You have reached the bottom, feeling completely relaxed and at ease.

Metaphors

Imagine yourself standing at the edge of a peaceful, calm river. The water flows gently, representing the passage of time. As you watch the water, you notice leaves floating on the surface, each leaf representing a memory or emotion. Some leaves are vibrant and beautiful, while others are wilted and faded, representing the pain and grief you have experienced.

As you observe the leaves, you realize that they are all part of the natural flow of life. Just as the river carries the leaves downstream, time carries your memories and emotions, allowing you to heal and grow.

Direct Suggestions

As you continue to relax, know that you have the ability to overcome grief and find healing. Each day, you are becoming more and more skilled at acknowledging your emotions and finding healthy ways to process them. You are able to honor the memories of those you have lost while also embracing the present and looking forward to the future.

Indirect Suggestions

You might find yourself discovering new ways to cope with grief, such as seeking support from friends and loved ones, engaging in activities that bring you joy, or finding solace in the beauty of nature. It's interesting how the mind can adapt and learn new techniques to heal and grow.

Embedded Commands

You can feel confident in your ability to overcome grief and find healing. Trust your inner strength to guide you through difficult times and remember that you are in control.

Post Hypnotic Suggestions

From this moment forward, whenever you feel grief beginning to surface, simply take a deep breath and remind yourself of your inner strength and ability to heal. You have the tools and resources to navigate the grieving process and find a sense of peace and acceptance.

Awakener

Now, it's time to return to full awareness. I will count from one to five, and with each number, you will become more and more awake, bringing with you the positive suggestions and feelings of relaxation.

1 - Beginning to awaken, feeling refreshed.
2 - Becoming more and more alert.
3 - Feeling your body and mind re-energize.
4 - Almost completely awake, feeling wonderful.
5 - Fully awake and alert, feeling refreshed and ready to face the day with a sense of healing and acceptance.

Take a moment to stretch and enjoy the feeling of relaxation and rejuvenation. Remember, you have the power to overcome grief and find healing in your life.

GRIEF SESSION 2

Pre-talk

Welcome to this hypnosis session designed to help you cope with grief and find inner strength. Before we begin, please make sure you are in a comfortable and quiet environment where you can fully relax without any interruptions. Ensure you are seated or lying down in a relaxed position. Remember, hypnosis is a natural state of focused relaxation, and you are always in control. This session aims to guide you in tapping into your own inner resources to effectively cope with grief.

Induction

Let's begin by finding a comfortable position, either sitting or lying down. Close your eyes and take a few slow, deep breaths. Inhale through your nose, and exhale through your mouth. With each breath, feel your body becoming more and more relaxed, allowing any tension or stress to simply dissipate.

As you continue to breathe, imagine a calming wave of relaxation gently washing over your body, starting at your head and gradually moving down to your toes. Feel this wave soothing every muscle, releasing any tension as it passes through.

Deepener

Now, picture yourself standing in a beautiful garden filled with colorful flowers and lush greenery. This garden represents your inner sanctuary, a place of peace and tranquility where you can find solace and healing.

As you walk through the garden, notice the gentle breeze caressing your skin, the warmth of the sun on your face, and the soothing sounds of nature around you. With each step, you feel more and more relaxed and at ease, allowing yourself to be fully present in this peaceful environment.

Metaphors

As you continue to explore the garden, you come across a beautiful butterfly resting on a flower. This butterfly represents transformation and growth. Just as the butterfly emerges from its cocoon, transformed and renewed, you too can emerge from your grief, stronger and more resilient.

Take a moment to observe the butterfly, admiring its delicate beauty and grace. As it takes flight, you realize that you have the ability to transform your grief into strength, allowing you to honor the memory of your loved one while also embracing the present and looking forward to the future.

Direct Suggestions

As you continue to relax, know that you possess the ability to cope with grief and find healing. Each day, you are becoming more skilled at recognizing and addressing your emotions, allowing yourself to process your grief in a healthy and constructive manner. You have the power to maintain a sense of balance and peace, no matter what challenges you may face.

Indirect Suggestions

It's amazing how the mind can develop new strategies for coping with grief, such as engaging in relaxation techniques, practicing mindfulness, or seeking support from friends and loved ones.

Embedded Commands

Trust in your inner strength and resilience to help you navigate through the grieving process.

Remember that you have the power to create a sense of balance and peace in your life.

Post Hypnotic Suggestions

From now on, whenever you feel grief beginning to build, take a moment to pause and remind yourself of your inner strength and resilience. You have the tools and resources necessary to effectively cope with grief and maintain a sense of balance in your life.

Awakener

It's time to return to full awareness. I will count from one to five, and with each number, you will become more and more awake, bringing with you the positive suggestions and feelings of relaxation.

1—Beginning to awaken, feeling rejuvenated.
2—Becoming more alert and aware.
3—Feeling your body and mind re-energize.
4—Almost completely awake, feeling refreshed and revitalized.
5—Fully awake and alert, ready to face the day with a renewed sense of strength and resilience.

Take a moment to stretch and enjoy the feeling of relaxation and rejuvenation. Remember, you

possess the power to cope with grief and find healing in your life.

RELEASE TRAUMA SESSION 1

Pre-talk

Welcome to this hypnosis session designed to help you release trauma and find healing. Before we begin, please ensure that you are in a comfortable and safe environment, free from any distractions. Make sure you are seated or lying down in a relaxed position. Remember, hypnosis is a natural state of relaxation and focus, and you are always in control. This session is about guiding you to discover your own inner resources for healing and moving forward.

Induction

Now, let's begin. Close your eyes and take a few deep breaths. Inhale through your nose, and exhale through your mouth. With each breath, feel your body becoming more and more relaxed. Allow any tension or stress to simply melt away as you focus on your breathing.

As you continue to breathe, I'd like you to imagine a warm, soothing light at the top of your head. This light represents relaxation and comfort. As this light begins to spread, feel the muscles in your forehead and face relax. Allow this warm light to continue spreading down to your neck and shoulders, releasing any tension that may be stored there.

Deepener

The soothing light continues to move down your arms, through your chest and stomach, and into your hips and legs. With each breath, this warm light is filling your body, leaving you completely relaxed and at ease.

Now, imagine yourself at the top of a staircase with ten steps. Each step represents a deeper level of relaxation. As I count down from ten to one, you will descend the staircase, feeling more and more relaxed with each step.

10 - Taking the first step, feeling more relaxed.
9 - Deeper and deeper.
8 - Feeling lighter and more at ease.
7 - Your body and mind are becoming one.
6 - Halfway there, feeling completely relaxed.
5 - Deeper still, as you continue to descend.
4 - Almost at the bottom, feeling so peaceful.
3 - Just a few more steps.
2 - At the edge of complete relaxation.

1 - You have reached the bottom, feeling completely relaxed and at ease.

Metaphors

Imagine yourself standing in a beautiful forest, surrounded by tall, strong trees. These trees represent your inner strength and resilience. As you walk through the forest, you notice a gentle stream flowing nearby. The water in the stream is crystal clear, symbolizing the cleansing and healing power of nature.

As you approach the stream, you notice that the water is gently washing away any debris and dirt, leaving the stones beneath it clean and smooth. This stream represents your ability to release trauma and cleanse your mind, body, and spirit.

Direct Suggestions

As you continue to relax, know that you have the ability to release trauma and find healing. Each day, you are becoming more and more skilled at acknowledging your emotions and finding healthy ways to process them. You are able to honor your experiences while also embracing the present and looking forward to the future.

Indirect Suggestions

You might find yourself discovering new ways to cope with trauma, such as seeking support from friends and loved ones, engaging in activities that bring you joy, or finding solace in the beauty of nature. It's interesting how the mind can adapt and learn new techniques to heal and grow.

Embedded Commands

You can feel confident in your ability to release trauma and find healing. Trust your inner strength to guide you through difficult times and remember that you are in control.

Post Hypnotic Suggestions

From this moment forward, whenever you feel the need to release trauma, simply take a deep breath and remind yourself of your inner strength and ability to heal. You have the tools and resources to navigate the healing process and find a sense of peace and acceptance.

Awakener

Now, it's time to return to full awareness. I will count from one to five, and with each number, you will become more and more awake, bringing with you the positive suggestions and feelings of relaxation.

1 - Beginning to awaken, feeling refreshed.
2 - Becoming more and more alert.
3 - Feeling your body and mind re-energize.
4 - Almost completely awake, feeling wonderful.
5 - Fully awake and alert, feeling refreshed and ready to face the day with a sense of healing and acceptance.

Take a moment to stretch and enjoy the feeling of relaxation and rejuvenation. Remember, you have the power to release trauma and find healing in your life.

RELEASE TRAUMA 2

Pre-talk

Welcome to this hypnosis session designed to help you release trauma and find inner healing. Before we begin, please make sure you are in a comfortable and quiet environment where you can fully relax without any interruptions. Ensure you are seated or lying down in a relaxed position. Remember, hypnosis is a natural state of focused relaxation, and you are always in control. This session aims to guide you in tapping into your own inner resources to effectively release trauma.

Induction

Let's begin by finding a comfortable position, either sitting or lying down. Close your eyes and take a few slow, deep breaths. Inhale through your nose, and exhale through your mouth. With each breath, feel your body becoming more and more relaxed, allowing any tension or stress to simply dissipate.

As you continue to breathe, imagine a calming wave of relaxation gently washing over your body, starting at your head and gradually moving down to your toes. Feel this wave soothing every muscle, releasing any tension as it passes through.

Deepener

Now, picture yourself standing on a beautiful beach, with soft, warm sand beneath your feet. The sound of the waves gently crashing on the shore and the warmth of the sun on your skin create a sense of peace and tranquility.

As you walk along the beach, you feel more and more relaxed, allowing yourself to be fully present in this serene environment. The soothing ocean breeze carries away any stress or tension, leaving you feeling completely at ease.

Metaphors

As you continue to walk along the beach, you notice a small, delicate shell lying in the sand. This shell represents your past experiences and the trauma you have faced. As you hold the shell in your hand, you realize that, just like the shell, you too have weathered the storms of life and have emerged stronger and more resilient.

You gently place the shell back on the sand, allowing the waves to wash over it, cleansing and purifying it. This symbolizes your ability to release the trauma from your past, allowing the healing power of nature to cleanse and renew your spirit.

Direct Suggestions

As you continue to relax, know that you possess the ability to release trauma and find healing. Each day, you are becoming more skilled at recognizing and addressing your emotions, allowing yourself to process your trauma in a healthy and constructive manner. You have the power to maintain a sense of balance and peace, no matter what challenges you may face.

Indirect Suggestions

It's amazing how the mind can develop new strategies for coping with trauma, such as engaging in relaxation techniques, practicing mindfulness, or seeking support from friends and loved ones.

Embedded Commands

Trust in your inner strength and resilience to help you navigate through the healing process.

Remember that you have the power to create a sense of balance and peace in your life.

Post Hypnotic Suggestions

From now on, whenever you feel the need to release trauma, take a moment to pause and remind yourself of your inner strength and resilience. You have the tools and resources necessary to effectively cope with trauma and maintain a sense of balance in your life.

Awakener

It's time to return to full awareness. I will count from one to five, and with each number, you will become more and more awake, bringing with you the positive suggestions and feelings of relaxation.

1 - Beginning to awaken, feeling rejuvenated.
2 - Becoming more alert and aware.
3 - Feeling your body and mind re-energize.
4 - Almost completely awake, feeling refreshed and revitalized.
5 - Fully awake and alert, ready to face the day with a renewed sense of strength and resilience.

Take a moment to stretch and enjoy the feeling of relaxation and rejuvenation. Remember, you

possess the power to release trauma and find healing in your life.

OVERCOMING ADDICTIONS 1

Pre-talk

Welcome to this hypnosis session designed to help you overcome harmful addictions. Before we begin, please ensure that you are in a comfortable and safe environment, free from any distractions. Make sure you are seated or lying down in a relaxed position. Remember, hypnosis is a natural state of relaxation and focus, and you are always in control. This session is about guiding you to discover your own inner resources for breaking free from addiction and regaining control over your life.

Induction

Now, let's begin. Close your eyes and take a few deep breaths. Inhale through your nose, and exhale through your mouth. With each breath, feel your body becoming more and more relaxed. Allow any tension or stress to simply melt away as you focus on your breathing.

As you continue to breathe, I'd like you to imagine a warm, soothing light at the top of your head. This light represents relaxation and comfort. As this light begins to spread, feel the muscles in your forehead and face relax. Allow this warm light to continue spreading down to your neck and shoulders, releasing any tension that may be stored there.

Deepener

The soothing light continues to move down your arms, through your chest and stomach, and into your hips and legs. With each breath, this warm light is filling your body, leaving you completely relaxed and at ease.

Now, imagine yourself at the top of a staircase with ten steps. Each step represents a deeper level of relaxation. As I count down from ten to one, you will descend the staircase, feeling more and more relaxed with each step.

10 - Taking the first step, feeling more relaxed.
9 - Deeper and deeper.
8 - Feeling lighter and more at ease.
7 - Your body and mind are becoming one.
6 - Halfway there, feeling completely relaxed.
5 - Deeper still, as you continue to descend.
4 - Almost at the bottom, feeling so peaceful.
3 - Just a few more steps.
2 - At the edge of complete relaxation.

1 - You have reached the bottom, feeling completely relaxed and at ease.

Metaphors

Imagine yourself standing in a beautiful garden filled with vibrant, healthy plants. These plants represent your inner strength, growth, and potential. As you walk through the garden, you notice a tangled, overgrown vine that represents your addiction.

With a pair of pruning shears in hand, you begin to carefully cut away the vine, symbolizing your commitment to overcoming addiction. As you remove the vine, the healthy plants beneath it are revealed, representing your true self, free from the constraints of addiction.

Direct Suggestions

As you continue to relax, know that you have the ability to overcome harmful addictions. Each day, you are becoming more and more skilled at recognizing triggers and finding healthy ways to cope. You are able to honor your experiences while also embracing the present and looking forward to a future free from addiction.

Indirect Suggestions

You might find yourself discovering new ways to cope with addiction, such as seeking support from friends and loved ones, engaging in activities that bring you joy, or finding solace in the beauty of nature. It's interesting how the mind can adapt and learn new techniques to heal and grow.

Embedded Commands

You can feel confident in your ability to overcome harmful addictions. Trust your inner strength to guide you through difficult times and remember that you are in control.

Post Hypnotic Suggestions

From this moment forward, whenever you feel the need to confront an addictive behavior, simply take a deep breath and remind yourself of your inner strength and ability to overcome. You have the tools and resources to navigate the healing process and find a sense of peace and freedom.

Awakener

Now, it's time to return to full awareness. I will count from one to five, and with each number, you will become more and more awake, bringing with you the positive suggestions and feelings of relaxation.

1 - Beginning to awaken, feeling refreshed.
2 - Becoming more and more alert.
3 - Feeling your body and mind re-energize.
4 - Almost completely awake, feeling wonderful.
5 - Fully awake and alert, feeling refreshed and ready to face the day with a sense of freedom and control over your life.

Take a moment to stretch and enjoy the feeling of relaxation and rejuvenation. Remember, you have the power to overcome harmful addictions and regain control over your life.

Overcoming Addiction 2

Pre-talk

Welcome to this hypnosis session designed to help you overcome harmful addictions. Before we begin, please ensure that you are in a comfortable and safe environment, free from any distractions. Make sure you are seated or lying down in a relaxed position. Remember, hypnosis is a natural state of relaxation and focus, and you are always in control. This session is about guiding you to discover your own inner resources for breaking free from addiction and creating a healthier, more balanced life.

Induction

Now, let's begin. Close your eyes and take a few deep breaths. Inhale through your nose, and exhale through your mouth. With each breath, feel your body becoming more and more relaxed. Allow any tension or stress to simply melt away as you focus on your breathing.

As you continue to breathe, I'd like you to imagine a gentle, calming breeze surrounding you. This breeze represents relaxation and comfort. As the breeze flows around you, feel the muscles in your forehead and face relax. Allow this calming breeze to continue flowing down to your neck and shoulders, releasing any tension that may be stored there.

Deepener

The soothing breeze continues to flow down your arms, through your chest and stomach, and into your hips and legs. With each breath, this calming breeze is filling your body, leaving you completely relaxed and at ease.

Now, imagine yourself standing in a peaceful forest. The sound of rustling leaves and the warmth of dappled sunlight create a sense of tranquility. As you walk through the forest, you feel more and more relaxed, allowing yourself to be fully present in this serene environment.

Metaphors

As you continue to walk through the forest, you notice a large boulder blocking your path. This boulder represents your addiction. With determination, you begin to push the boulder, symbolizing your commitment to overcoming addiction. As you push, the boulder starts to crumble and eventually breaks apart, revealing a clear path ahead, representing your true self, free from the constraints of addiction.

Direct Suggestions

As you continue to relax, know that you have the ability to overcome harmful addictions. Each day, you are becoming more and more skilled at recognizing triggers and finding healthy ways to cope. You are able to honor your experiences while also embracing the present and looking forward to a future free from addiction.

Indirect Suggestions

It's fascinating how the mind can develop new strategies for coping with addiction, such as engaging in relaxation techniques, practicing mindfulness, or seeking support from friends and loved ones.

Embedded Commands

Believe in your inner strength and resilience to help you navigate through the healing process.

Remember that you have the power to create a sense of balance and peace in your life.

Post Hypnotic Suggestions

From now on, whenever you feel the need to address an addictive behavior, take a moment to pause and remind yourself of your inner strength and resilience. You have the tools and resources necessary to effectively cope with addiction and maintain a sense of balance in your life.

Awakener

It's time to return to full awareness. I will count from one to five, and with each number, you will become more and more awake, bringing with you the positive suggestions and feelings of relaxation.

1 - Beginning to awaken, feeling rejuvenated.
2 - Becoming more alert and aware.
3 - Feeling your body and mind re-energize.
4 - Almost completely awake, feeling refreshed and revitalized.
5 - Fully awake and alert, ready to face the day with a renewed sense of strength and resilience.

Take a moment to stretch and enjoy the feeling of relaxation and rejuvenation. Remember, you

possess the power to overcome harmful addictions and create a healthier, more balanced life.

ATTRACTING ABUNDANCE 1

Pre-talk

Welcome to this hypnosis session designed to help you attract abundance into your life. Before we begin, please ensure that you are in a comfortable and safe environment, free from any distractions. Make sure you are seated or lying down in a relaxed position. Remember, hypnosis is a natural state of relaxation and focus, and you are always in control. This session is about guiding you to discover your own inner resources for manifesting abundance and creating a fulfilling life.

Induction

Now, let's begin. Close your eyes and take a few deep breaths. Inhale through your nose, and exhale through your mouth. With each breath, feel your body becoming more and more relaxed. Allow any tension or stress to simply melt away as you focus on your breathing.

As you continue to breathe, I'd like you to imagine a warm, golden light at the top of your head. This light represents abundance and prosperity. As this light begins to spread, feel the muscles in your forehead and face relax. Allow this warm, golden light to continue spreading down to your neck and shoulders, releasing any tension that may be stored there.

Deepener

The soothing light continues to move down your arms, through your chest and stomach, and into your hips and legs. With each breath, this warm, golden light is filling your body, leaving you completely relaxed and at ease.

Now, imagine yourself standing at the top of a beautiful hill. As you look around, you see a vast landscape filled with lush, green fields, sparkling rivers, and thriving forests. This landscape represents the abundance that surrounds you. As you begin to walk down the hill, feel yourself becoming more and more relaxed, fully embracing this abundant environment.

Metaphors

As you walk through this landscape, you come across a magnificent tree with golden leaves. This tree represents your inner wealth and abundance. As you approach the tree, you notice that some of the golden leaves are falling to the ground, symbolizing the abundance that is available to you.

You reach out and pick up a handful of golden leaves, feeling their warmth and energy. You understand that these leaves represent the opportunities and resources that are available to you, and you feel a deep sense of gratitude for this abundance.

Direct Suggestions

As you continue to relax, know that you have the ability to attract abundance into your life. Each day, you are becoming more and more skilled at recognizing opportunities and resources that can help you create a fulfilling life. You are able to honor your experiences while also embracing the present and looking forward to a future filled with abundance and prosperity.

Indirect Suggestions

You might find yourself discovering new ways to attract abundance, such as setting clear intentions, practicing gratitude, or seeking support from friends and loved ones. It's interesting how the mind can adapt and learn new techniques to manifest abundance and create a fulfilling life.

Embedded Commands

You can feel confident in your ability to attract abundance. Trust your inner wisdom to guide you toward opportunities and resources that can help you create a prosperous life.

Post Hypnotic Suggestions

From this moment forward, whenever you feel the need to tap into your inner abundance, simply take a deep breath and remind yourself of the golden leaves that symbolize the wealth and prosperity that surrounds you. You have the tools and resources to manifest abundance and create a fulfilling life.

Awakener

Now, it's time to return to full awareness. I will count from one to five, and with each number, you will become more and more awake, bringing with you the positive suggestions and feelings of relaxation.

1 - Beginning to awaken, feeling refreshed.
2 - Becoming more and more alert.
3 - Feeling your body and mind re-energize.
4 - Almost completely awake, feeling wonderful.
5 - Fully awake and alert, feeling refreshed and

ready to face the day with a sense of abundance and prosperity.

Take a moment to stretch and enjoy the feeling of relaxation and rejuvenation. Remember, you have the power to attract abundance and create a fulfilling life.

ATTRACT ABUNDANCE 2

Pre-talk

Welcome to this hypnosis session designed to help you attract abundance into your life. Before we begin, please ensure that you are in a comfortable and safe environment, free from any distractions. Make sure you are seated or lying down in a relaxed position. Remember, hypnosis is a natural state of relaxation and focus, and you are always in control. This session is about guiding you to discover your own inner resources for manifesting abundance and creating a life of prosperity and fulfillment.

Induction

Now, let's begin. Close your eyes and take a few deep breaths. Inhale through your nose, and exhale through your mouth. With each breath, feel your body becoming more and more relaxed. Allow any tension or stress to simply melt away as you focus on your breathing.

As you continue to breathe, I'd like you to imagine a gentle, soothing waterfall cascading down from above. This waterfall represents the flow of abundance and prosperity. As the water gently touches your head, feel the muscles in your forehead and face relax. Allow this soothing waterfall to continue flowing down your neck and shoulders, releasing any tension that may be stored there.

Deepener

The calming waterfall continues to flow down your arms, through your chest and stomach, and into your hips and legs. With each breath, this soothing waterfall is filling your body, leaving you completely relaxed and at ease.

Now, imagine yourself standing in a lush, abundant garden. The vibrant colors and fragrances of the flowers and plants surrounding you create a sense of tranquility and peace. As you walk through the garden, you feel more and more relaxed, allowing yourself to be fully present in this abundant environment.

Metaphors

As you continue to explore the garden, you come across a beautiful, crystal-clear pond. This pond represents the abundance that is available to you. You notice that the water in the pond is filled with shimmering, golden coins, symbolizing wealth and prosperity.

You reach into the pond and pick up a handful of golden coins, feeling their weight and energy. You understand that these coins represent the opportunities and resources that are available to you, and you feel a deep sense of gratitude for this abundance.

Direct Suggestions

As you continue to relax, know that you have the ability to attract abundance into your life. Each day, you are becoming more and more skilled at recognizing opportunities and resources that can help you create a prosperous and fulfilling life. You are able to honor your experiences while also embracing the present and looking forward to a future filled with abundance and success.

Indirect Suggestions

It's fascinating how the mind can develop new strategies for attracting abundance, such as visualizing success, practicing gratitude, or connecting with like-minded individuals who share your goals and aspirations.

Embedded Commands

Believe in your inner strength and ability to attract abundance. Trust your intuition to guide you toward opportunities and resources that can help you create a prosperous life.

Post Hypnotic Suggestions

From now on, whenever you need to tap into your inner abundance, simply take a moment to pause and remind yourself of the shimmering golden coins that symbolize the wealth and prosperity that surrounds you. You have the tools and resources necessary to effectively manifest abundance and create a life of prosperity and fulfillment.

Awakener

It's time to return to full awareness. I will count from one to five, and with each number, you will become more and more awake, bringing with you the positive suggestions and feelings of relaxation.

1 - Beginning to awaken, feeling rejuvenated.
2 - Becoming more alert and aware.
3 - Feeling your body and mind re-energize.
4 - Almost completely awake, feeling refreshed and revitalized.

5 - Fully awake and alert, ready to face the day with a renewed sense of abundance and prosperity.

Take a moment to stretch and enjoy the feeling of relaxation and rejuvenation. Remember, you possess the power to attract abundance and create a prosperous, fulfilling life.

CONFIDENCE BUILDING EGO STRENGTHENING 1

Pre-talk

Welcome to this hypnosis session designed to help you build self-confidence and a strong sense of self. Before we begin, please ensure that you are in a comfortable and safe environment, free from any distractions. Make sure you are seated or lying down in a relaxed position. Remember, hypnosis is a natural state of relaxation and focus, and you are always in control. This session is about guiding you to discover your own inner resources for developing a healthy self-image and empowering belief in yourself.

Induction

Now, let's begin. Close your eyes and take a few deep breaths. Inhale through your nose, and exhale through your mouth. With each breath, feel your body becoming more and more relaxed. Allow any tension or stress to simply melt away as you focus on your breathing.

As you continue to breathe, I'd like you to imagine a bright, radiant light at the center of your chest. This light represents your inner strength and self-confidence. As this light begins to grow, feel the muscles in your chest and shoulders relax. Allow this warm, radiant light to continue spreading throughout your body, releasing any tension that may be stored.

Deepener

The soothing light continues to move through your arms, down your spine, and into your hips and legs. With each breath, this warm, radiant light is filling your body, leaving you completely relaxed and at ease.

Now, imagine yourself standing at the edge of a beautiful, calm lake. The stillness of the water reflects a sense of inner peace and tranquility. As you gaze at the lake, you feel more and more relaxed, fully embracing this serene environment.

Metaphors

As you walk along the shore, you notice a small, sturdy boat waiting for you. This boat represents your journey toward self-confidence and a strong sense of self. You step into the boat and begin to row, moving smoothly and effortlessly through the calm waters.

As you row, you notice that with each stroke, your confidence grows stronger, and your belief in yourself becomes more unwavering. The boat continues to glide through the water, symbolizing your journey toward self-empowerment and inner strength.

Direct Suggestions

As you continue to relax, know that you have the ability to cultivate self-confidence and a strong sense of self. Each day, you are becoming more and more skilled at recognizing your own worth and embracing your unique qualities. You are able to honor your experiences while also embracing the present and looking forward to a future filled with self-belief and personal growth.

Indirect Suggestions

You might find yourself discovering new ways to develop self-confidence, such as setting achievable goals, practicing self-compassion, or seeking support from friends and loved ones. It's interesting how the mind can adapt and learn new techniques to cultivate a healthy self-image and empowering belief in oneself.

Embedded Commands

You can feel confident in your ability to build self-confidence and a strong sense of self. Trust your inner wisdom to guide you toward opportunities and experiences that can help you grow and develop as an individual.

Post Hypnotic Suggestions

From this moment forward, whenever you need to remind yourself of your inner strength and self-confidence, simply take a deep breath and recall the radiant light at the center of your chest. You have the tools and resources to cultivate a healthy self-image and empowering belief in yourself.

Awakener

Now, it's time to return to full awareness. I will count from one to five, and with each number, you will become more and more awake, bringing with you the positive suggestions and feelings of relaxation.

1 - Beginning to awaken, feeling refreshed.
2 - Becoming more and more alert.
3 - Feeling your body and mind re-energize.
4 - Almost completely awake, feeling wonderful.

5 - Fully awake and alert, feeling refreshed and ready to face the day with a renewed sense of self-confidence and inner strength.

Take a moment to stretch and enjoy the feeling of relaxation and rejuvenation. Remember, you have the power to cultivate self-confidence and a strong sense of self, empowering you to live a fulfilling life.

CONFIDENCE BUILDING EGO STRENGTHENING 2

Pre-talk

Welcome to this hypnosis session designed to help you enhance your self-assurance and inner resilience. Before we begin, please ensure that you are in a comfortable and safe environment, free from any distractions. Make sure you are seated or lying down in a relaxed position. Remember, hypnosis is a natural state of relaxation and focus, and you are always in control. This session is about guiding you to discover your own inner resources for developing a positive self-image and unwavering faith in your abilities.

Induction

Now, let's begin. Close your eyes and take a few deep breaths. Inhale through your nose, and exhale through your mouth. With each breath, feel your body becoming more and more relaxed. Allow any

tension or stress to simply melt away as you focus on your breathing.

As you continue to breathe, I'd like you to imagine a powerful, protective shield surrounding your entire body. This shield represents your inner resilience and self-assurance. As the shield forms around you, feel the muscles in your body relax, and allow this shield to protect you from any negative thoughts or doubts.

Deepener

The protective shield continues to surround you, providing a sense of safety and comfort. With each breath, you feel more relaxed and at ease, fully embracing this nurturing environment.

Now, imagine yourself walking through a tranquil forest. The tall trees and lush foliage create a sense of peace and calm. As you walk through the forest, you feel more and more relaxed, allowing yourself to be fully present in this serene environment.

Metaphors

As you continue to explore the forest, you come across a clear, sparkling stream. This stream represents the flow of positive energy and self-assurance. You notice that the water in the stream is filled with shimmering, silver light, symbolizing your inner resilience and strength.

You reach into the stream and cup your hands, gathering the shimmering, silver light. As you hold this light, you understand that it represents your innate ability to cultivate self-assurance and inner resilience. You feel a deep sense of gratitude for this inner strength.

Direct Suggestions

As you continue to relax, know that you have the ability to enhance your self-assurance and inner resilience. Each day, you are becoming more and more skilled at recognizing your own value and embracing your unique strengths. You are able to honor your experiences while also embracing the present and looking forward to a future filled with self-belief and personal growth.

Indirect Suggestions

It's fascinating how the mind can develop new strategies for enhancing self-assurance, such as focusing on accomplishments, practicing self-compassion, or connecting with supportive individuals who share your goals and aspirations.

Embedded Commands

Believe in your inner strength and ability to enhance your self-assurance and inner resilience. Trust your intuition to guide you toward opportunities and experiences that can help you grow and develop as an individual.

Post Hypnotic Suggestions

From now on, whenever you need to remind yourself of your inner resilience and self-assurance, simply take a moment to pause and recall the shimmering, silver light that symbolizes your strength and ability to overcome challenges. You have the tools and resources necessary to effectively enhance your self-assurance and inner resilience.

Awakener

It's time to return to full awareness. I will count from one to five, and with each number, you will become more and more awake, bringing with you the positive suggestions and feelings of relaxation.

1 - Beginning to awaken, feeling rejuvenated.
2 - Becoming more alert and aware.
3 - Feeling your body and mind re-energize.
4 - Almost completely awake, feeling refreshed and

revitalized.
5 - Fully awake and alert, ready to face the day with a renewed sense of self-assurance and inner resilience.

Take a moment to stretch and enjoy the feeling of relaxation and rejuvenation. Remember, you possess the power to enhance your self-assurance and inner resilience, empowering you to live a fulfilling life.

RELEASING ANGER 1

Pre-talk

Welcome to this hypnosis session designed to help you release anger and embrace inner peace. Before we begin, please ensure that you are in a comfortable and safe environment, free from any distractions. Make sure you are seated or lying down in a relaxed position. Remember, hypnosis is a natural state of relaxation and focus, and you are always in control. This session is about guiding you to discover your own inner resources for letting go of anger and cultivating a sense of calm and tranquility.

Induction

Now, let's begin. Close your eyes and take a few deep breaths. Inhale through your nose, and exhale through your mouth. With each breath, feel your body becoming more and more relaxed. Allow any tension or stress to simply melt away as you focus on your breathing.

As you continue to breathe, I'd like you to imagine a warm, soothing light enveloping your entire body. This light represents a sense of peace and calm. As the light surrounds you, feel the muscles in your body relax, and allow this warm, soothing light to release any tension that may be stored.

Deepener

The calming light continues to move through your body, from your head down to your toes. With each breath, this warm, soothing light is filling your body, leaving you completely relaxed and at ease.

Now, imagine yourself walking along a beautiful, serene beach. The sound of the waves crashing against the shore and the feeling of the warm sand beneath your feet create a sense of tranquility and peace. As you walk along the beach, you feel more and more relaxed, fully embracing this calming environment.

Metaphors

As you continue to walk along the shore, you notice a large, heavy stone. This stone represents the anger and frustration that you have been holding onto. You pick up the stone and feel its weight, acknowledging the burden that this anger has placed upon you.

You then look out at the vast, open ocean and realize that you have the power to release this anger. You take a deep breath and, with all your strength, you throw the stone into the ocean, watching as it sinks beneath the waves and disappears from view.

Direct Suggestions

As you continue to relax, know that you have the ability to release anger and embrace inner peace. Each day, you are becoming more and more skilled at recognizing and addressing the emotions that may be causing you distress. You are able to honor your experiences while also embracing the present and looking forward to a future filled with peace and tranquility.

Indirect Suggestions

You might find yourself discovering new ways to release anger, such as practicing mindfulness, engaging in physical activity, or seeking support from friends and loved ones. It's interesting how the mind can adapt and learn new techniques to let go of negative emotions and cultivate a sense of calm and tranquility.

Embedded Commands

Trust in your inner strength and ability to release anger and embrace inner peace. Allow your intuition to guide you toward opportunities and experiences that can help you cultivate a sense of calm and tranquility.

Post Hypnotic Suggestions

From this moment forward, whenever you need to release anger and embrace inner peace, simply take a deep breath and recall the image of the heavy stone being thrown into the ocean. You have the tools and resources necessary to effectively let go of anger and cultivate a sense of calm and tranquility.

Awakener

Now, it's time to return to full awareness. I will count from one to five, and with each number, you will become more and more awake, bringing with you the positive suggestions and feelings of relaxation.

1 - Beginning to awaken, feeling refreshed.
2 - Becoming more and more alert.
3 - Feeling your body and mind re-energize.
4 - Almost completely awake, feeling rejuvenated.
5 - Fully awake and alert, ready to face the day with a renewed sense of inner peace and tranquility.

Take a moment to stretch and enjoy the feeling of relaxation and rejuvenation. Remember, you have the power to release anger and embrace inner peace, empowering you to live a fulfilling and harmonious life.

RELEASING ANGER 2

Pre-talk

Welcome to this hypnosis session designed to help you let go of anger and foster a sense of inner harmony. Before we begin, please ensure that you are in a comfortable and safe environment, free from any distractions. Make sure you are seated or lying down in a relaxed position. Remember, hypnosis is a natural state of relaxation and focus, and you are always in control. This session is about guiding you to discover your own inner resources for releasing anger and cultivating a sense of balance and tranquility.

Induction

Now, let's begin. Close your eyes and take a few deep breaths. Inhale through your nose, and exhale through your mouth. With each breath, feel your body becoming more and more relaxed. Allow any tension or stress to simply melt away as you focus on your breathing.

As you continue to breathe, I'd like you to imagine a gentle, cool breeze caressing your entire body. This breeze represents a sense of calm and serenity. As the breeze flows around you, feel the muscles in your body relax, and allow this gentle, cool breeze to release any tension that may be stored.

Deepener

The soothing breeze continues to flow through your body, from your head down to your toes. With each breath, this gentle, cool breeze is filling your body, leaving you completely relaxed and at ease.

Now, imagine yourself standing at the top of a beautiful, lush hillside. The panoramic view of the landscape and the feeling of the soft grass beneath your feet create a sense of tranquility and peace. As you stand on the hillside, you feel more and more relaxed, fully embracing this calming environment.

Metaphors

As you continue to stand on the hillside, you notice a cluster of balloons tied together. Each balloon represents a different aspect of the anger and frustration that you have been holding onto. You take hold of the balloons and feel their weight, acknowledging the burden that this anger has placed upon you.

You then look up at the vast, open sky and realize that you have the power to release this anger. You take a deep breath and, with a sense of determination, you let go of the balloons, watching as they float away into the sky, becoming smaller and smaller until they disappear from view.

Direct Suggestions

As you continue to relax, know that you have the ability to let go of anger and foster a sense of inner harmony. Each day, you are becoming more and more skilled at recognizing and addressing the emotions that may be causing you distress. You are able to honor your experiences while also embracing the present and looking forward to a future filled with balance and tranquility.

Indirect Suggestions

It's fascinating how the mind can develop new strategies for letting go of anger, such as practicing meditation, engaging in creative expression, or connecting with supportive individuals who share your goals and aspirations.

Embedded Commands

Believe in your inner strength and ability to let go of anger and foster a sense of inner harmony. Allow your intuition to guide you toward opportunities and experiences that can help you cultivate a sense of balance and tranquility.

Post Hypnotic Suggestions

From now on, whenever you need to let go of anger and foster a sense of inner harmony, simply take a moment to pause and recall the image of the balloons floating away into the sky. You have the tools and resources necessary to effectively release anger and cultivate a sense of balance and tranquility.

Awakener

It's time to return to full awareness. I will count from one to five, and with each number, you will become more and more awake, bringing with you the positive suggestions and feelings of relaxation.

1 - Beginning to awaken, feeling rejuvenated.
2 - Becoming more alert and aware.
3 - Feeling your body and mind re-energize.
4 - Almost completely awake, feeling refreshed and revitalized.
5 - Fully awake and alert, ready to face the day with a renewed sense of inner harmony and tranquility.

Take a moment to stretch and enjoy the feeling of relaxation and rejuvenation. Remember, you possess the power to let go of anger and foster a sense of inner harmony, empowering you to live a fulfilling and balanced life.

OVERCOMING ADVERSITY 1

Pre-talk

Welcome to this hypnotic journey designed to guide you toward embracing your full potential and navigating through challenges with ease and confidence. Before we begin, please ensure that you are in a comfortable and safe environment, free from any distractions. Make sure you are seated or lying down in a relaxed position. Remember, hypnosis is a natural state of relaxation and focus, and you are always in control. This session is about guiding you to discover your own inner resources for enhancing your abilities and achieving success with grace.

Induction

As you begin to settle into a comfortable position, allow your eyes to gently close and take a few deep breaths. Inhale through your nose, and exhale through your mouth. With each breath, feel your body becoming more and more relaxed. Allow any tension or stress to simply melt away as you focus on your breathing.

As you continue to breathe, imagine a warm, golden light surrounding your entire body. This light represents a sense of calm and focus. As the light envelops you, feel the muscles in your body relax, and allow this warm, golden light to release any tension that may be stored.

Deepener

The soothing light continues to move through your body, from your head down to your toes. With each breath, this warm, golden light is filling your body, leaving you completely relaxed and at ease.

Now, imagine yourself in a beautiful, tranquil garden. The vibrant colors of the flowers and the gentle rustle of the leaves create a sense of peace and serenity. As you explore the garden, you feel more and more relaxed, fully embracing this calming environment.

Metaphors

As you continue to walk through the garden, you come across a magnificent tree. This tree represents the knowledge and wisdom that you have within you. You notice that the tree has strong roots that reach deep into the ground, symbolizing your solid foundation and ability to grow and adapt.

You reach out and touch the trunk of the tree, feeling a surge of energy and understanding. With this connection, you realize that you have the power to harness your full potential and achieve success with ease and confidence.

Direct Suggestions

As you continue to relax, know that you have the ability to enhance your abilities and navigate through challenges with grace. Each day, you are becoming more and more skilled at recognizing your strengths and embracing your unique capabilities. You are able to honor your experiences while also embracing the present and looking forward to a future filled with success and accomplishment.

Indirect Suggestions

You might find it interesting how the mind can develop new strategies for becoming more proficient and confident, such as setting realistic goals, practicing effective time management, or seeking guidance from knowledgeable individuals who share your aspirations.

Embedded Commands

Trust in your inner strength and ability to harness your full potential and achieve success with ease and confidence. Allow your intuition to guide you toward opportunities and experiences that can help you grow and develop as an individual.

Post Hypnotic Suggestions

From this moment forward, whenever you need to remind yourself of your ability to enhance your capabilities and navigate through challenges with grace, simply take a moment to pause and recall the image of the magnificent tree that symbolizes your knowledge and wisdom. You have the tools and resources necessary to effectively achieve success and accomplish your goals.

Awakener

Now, it's time to return to full awareness. I will count from one to five, and with each number, you will become more and more awake, bringing with you the positive suggestions and feelings of relaxation.

1 - Beginning to awaken, feeling rejuvenated.
2 - Becoming more alert and aware.
3 - Feeling your body and mind re-energize.
4 - Almost completely awake, feeling refreshed and revitalized.

5 - Fully awake and alert, ready to face the day with a renewed sense of confidence and ability.

Take a moment to stretch and enjoy the feeling of relaxation and rejuvenation. Remember, you possess the power to harness your full potential and achieve success with ease and grace, empowering you to live a fulfilling and accomplished life.

OVERCOMING ADVERSITY 2

Pre-talk

Welcome to this hypnotic journey designed to guide you toward embracing resilience and overcoming adversity with courage and determination. Before we begin, please ensure that you are in a comfortable and safe environment, free from any distractions. Make sure you are seated or lying down in a relaxed position. Remember, hypnosis is a natural state of relaxation and focus, and you are always in control. This session is about guiding you to discover your own inner resources for facing challenges and cultivating a sense of strength and perseverance.

Induction

As you begin to settle into a comfortable position, allow your eyes to gently close and take a few deep breaths. Inhale through your nose, and exhale through your mouth. With each breath, feel your body becoming more and more relaxed. Allow any tension or stress to simply melt away as you focus on your breathing.

As you continue to breathe, imagine a soft, nurturing light surrounding your entire body. This light represents a sense of calm and courage. As the light envelops you, feel the muscles in your body relax, and allow this soft, nurturing light to release any tension that may be stored.

Deepener

The comforting light continues to move through your body, from your head down to your toes. With each breath, this soft, nurturing light is filling your body, leaving you completely relaxed and at ease.

Now, imagine yourself standing at the edge of a beautiful, serene forest. The sounds of the rustling leaves and the gentle breeze create a sense of peace and tranquility. As you enter the forest, you feel more and more relaxed, fully embracing this calming environment.

Metaphors

As you continue to walk through the forest, you come across a winding path that leads up a hill. This path represents the journey of overcoming adversity. You notice that the path is filled with obstacles such as rocks, fallen branches, and steep inclines. These obstacles symbolize the challenges that you may encounter in life.

With determination and courage, you begin to navigate the path, overcoming each obstacle with grace and resilience. As you reach the top of the hill, you are filled with a sense of accomplishment and strength, knowing that you have the power to face any challenge that may come your way.

Direct Suggestions

As you continue to relax, know that you have the ability to overcome adversity with courage and determination. Each day, you are becoming more and more skilled at recognizing your strengths and embracing your unique capabilities. You are able to honor your experiences while also embracing the present and looking forward to a future filled with resilience and perseverance.

Indirect Suggestions

You might find it fascinating how the mind can develop new strategies for overcoming adversity, such as seeking support from others, practicing self-compassion, or focusing on personal growth and development.

Embedded Commands

Believe in your inner strength and ability to face challenges with courage and determination. Allow your intuition to guide you toward opportunities and experiences that can help you cultivate a sense of resilience and perseverance.

Post Hypnotic Suggestions

From this moment forward, whenever you need to remind yourself of your ability to overcome adversity, simply take a moment to pause and recall the image of the winding path that leads up the hill. You have the tools and resources necessary to effectively face challenges and cultivate a sense of strength and perseverance.

Awakener

Now, it's time to return to full awareness. I will count from one to five, and with each number, you will become more and more awake, bringing with you the positive suggestions and feelings of relaxation.

1 - Beginning to awaken, feeling rejuvenated.
2 - Becoming more alert and aware.
3 - Feeling your body and mind re-energize.
4 - Almost completely awake, feeling refreshed and revitalized.

5 - Fully awake and alert, ready to face the day with a renewed sense of courage and determination.

Take a moment to stretch and enjoy the feeling of relaxation and rejuvenation. Remember, you possess the power to overcome adversity with courage and determination, empowering you to live a fulfilling and resilient life.

FINDING INSPIRATION 1

Pre-talk

Welcome to this hypnotic journey designed to guide you toward discovering and embracing inspiration in your life. Before we begin, please ensure that you are in a comfortable and safe environment, free from any distractions. Make sure you are seated or lying down in a relaxed position. Remember, hypnosis is a natural state of relaxation and focus, and you are always in control. This session is about guiding you to discover your own inner resources for finding inspiration and cultivating a sense of creativity and passion.

Induction

As you begin to settle into a comfortable position, allow your eyes to gently close and take a few deep breaths. Inhale through your nose, and exhale through your mouth. With each breath, feel your body becoming more and more relaxed. Allow any

tension or stress to simply melt away as you focus on your breathing.

As you continue to breathe, imagine a radiant, shimmering light surrounding your entire body. This light represents a sense of creativity and inspiration. As the light envelops you, feel the muscles in your body relax, and allow this radiant, shimmering light to release any tension that may be stored.

Deepener

The invigorating light continues to move through your body, from your head down to your toes. With each breath, this radiant, shimmering light is filling your body, leaving you completely relaxed and at ease.

Now, imagine yourself standing at the entrance of a beautiful, enchanting garden. The vibrant colors of the flowers and the gentle sounds of nature create a sense of peace and wonder. As you explore the garden, you feel more and more relaxed, fully embracing this magical environment.

Metaphors

As you continue to walk through the garden, you come across a magnificent fountain. This fountain represents the wellspring of inspiration within you. You notice that the water in the fountain is shimmering with a multitude of colors, symbolizing the diverse sources of inspiration that you have within you.

You reach out and touch the water, feeling a surge of creativity and passion. With this connection, you realize that you have the power to tap into your own wellspring of inspiration, allowing you to cultivate a sense of wonder and creativity in your life.

Direct Suggestions

As you continue to relax, know that you have the ability to find inspiration and embrace your creativity. Each day, you are becoming more and more skilled at recognizing the diverse sources of inspiration that surround you. You are able to honor your experiences while also embracing the present and looking forward to a future filled with creativity and passion.

Indirect Suggestions

It's interesting how the mind can develop new strategies for finding inspiration, such as exploring new environments, engaging in creative activities, or connecting with others who share your interests and passions.

Embedded Commands

Trust in your inner strength and ability to tap into your wellspring of inspiration and embrace your creativity. Allow your intuition to guide you toward opportunities and experiences that can help you cultivate a sense of wonder and passion.

Post Hypnotic Suggestions

From this moment forward, whenever you need to remind yourself of your ability to find inspiration, simply take a moment to pause and recall the image of the magnificent fountain that symbolizes your wellspring of creativity. You have the tools and resources necessary to effectively discover and embrace inspiration in your life.

Awakener

Now, it's time to return to full awareness. I will count from one to five, and with each number, you will become more and more awake, bringing with you the positive suggestions and feelings of relaxation.

1 - Beginning to awaken, feeling rejuvenated.
2 - Becoming more alert and aware.
3 - Feeling your body and mind re-energize.
4 - Almost completely awake, feeling refreshed and revitalized.
5 - Fully awake and alert, ready to face the day with a renewed sense of creativity and inspiration.

Take a moment to stretch and enjoy the feeling of relaxation and rejuvenation. Remember, you possess the power to tap into your wellspring of inspiration, empowering you to live a fulfilling and creative life.

FINDING INSPIRATION 2

Pre-talk

Welcome to this hypnotic journey designed to guide you toward unlocking and embracing inspiration in your life. Before we begin, please ensure that you are in a comfortable and safe environment, free from any distractions. Make sure you are seated or lying down in a relaxed position. Remember, hypnosis is a natural state of relaxation and focus, and you are always in control. This session is about guiding you to discover your own inner resources for finding inspiration and nurturing a sense of creativity and passion.

Induction

As you begin to settle into a comfortable position, allow your eyes to gently close and take a few deep breaths. Inhale through your nose, and exhale through your mouth. With each breath, feel your body becoming more and more relaxed. Allow any

tension or stress to simply melt away as you focus on your breathing.

As you continue to breathe, imagine a soothing, warm light surrounding your entire body. This light represents a sense of creativity and inspiration. As the light envelops you, feel the muscles in your body relax, and allow this soothing, warm light to release any tension that may be stored.

Deepener

The calming light continues to move through your body, from your head down to your toes. With each breath, this soothing, warm light is filling your body, leaving you completely relaxed and at ease.

Now, imagine yourself standing at the edge of a serene, peaceful beach. The gentle sound of the waves and the warmth of the sun create a sense of tranquility and wonder. As you walk along the beach, you feel more and more relaxed, fully embracing this soothing environment.

Metaphors

As you continue to walk along the beach, you come across a beautiful seashell. This seashell represents the hidden treasures of inspiration within you. You notice that the seashell has intricate patterns and a unique shape, symbolizing the diverse sources of inspiration that you have within you.

You pick up the seashell and hold it in your hand, feeling a surge of creativity and passion. With this connection, you realize that you have the power to uncover your own hidden treasures of inspiration, allowing you to nurture a sense of wonder and creativity in your life.

Direct Suggestions

As you continue to relax, know that you have the ability to find inspiration and embrace your creativity. Each day, you are becoming more and more skilled at recognizing the diverse sources of inspiration that surround you. You are able to honor your experiences while also embracing the present and looking forward to a future filled with creativity and passion.

Indirect Suggestions

You might find it intriguing how the mind can develop new strategies for finding inspiration, such as immersing yourself in art, literature, or music, engaging in mindfulness practices, or seeking out new experiences that challenge and inspire you.

Embedded Commands

Believe in your inner strength and ability to uncover your hidden treasures of inspiration and embrace your creativity. Allow your intuition to guide you toward opportunities and experiences that can help you cultivate a sense of wonder and passion.

Post Hypnotic Suggestions

From this moment forward, whenever you need to remind yourself of your ability to find inspiration, simply take a moment to pause and recall the image of the beautiful seashell that symbolizes your hidden treasures of creativity. You have the tools and resources necessary to effectively discover and embrace inspiration in your life.

Awakener

Now, it's time to return to full awareness. I will count from one to five, and with each number, you will become more and more awake, bringing with you the positive suggestions and feelings of relaxation.

1 - Beginning to awaken, feeling rejuvenated.
2 - Becoming more alert and aware.
3 - Feeling your body and mind re-energize.

4 - Almost completely awake, feeling refreshed and revitalized.
5 - Fully awake and alert, ready to face the day with a renewed sense of creativity and inspiration.

Take a moment to stretch and enjoy the feeling of relaxation and rejuvenation. Remember, you possess the power to uncover your hidden treasures of inspiration, empowering you to live a fulfilling and creative life.

THIRD EYE 1

Pre-talk

Welcome to this hypnotic journey designed to guide you toward opening up your intuitive center, enhancing your perception and awareness beyond the physical senses. Before we begin, please ensure that you are in a comfortable and safe environment, free from any distractions. Make sure you are seated or lying down in a relaxed position. Remember, hypnosis is a natural state of relaxation and focus, and you are always in control. This session is about guiding you to discover your own inner resources for expanding your consciousness and connecting with your innate intuition.

Induction

As you begin to settle into a comfortable position, allow your eyes to gently close and take a few deep breaths. Inhale through your nose, and exhale through your mouth. With each breath, feel your body becoming more and more relaxed. Allow any tension or stress to simply melt away as you focus on your breathing.

As you continue to breathe, imagine a soothing, gentle light surrounding your entire body. This light represents a sense of calm and inner wisdom. As the light envelops you, feel the muscles in your body relax, and allow this soothing, gentle light to release any tension that may be stored.

Deepener

The calming light continues to move through your body, from your head down to your toes. With each breath, this soothing, gentle light is filling your body, leaving you completely relaxed and at ease.

Now, imagine yourself standing at the entrance of a beautiful, ancient temple. The intricate architecture and the serene atmosphere create a sense of peace and reverence. As you explore the temple, you feel more and more relaxed, fully embracing this sacred environment.

Metaphors

As you continue to walk through the temple, you come across a magnificent crystal, glowing with a soft, radiant light. This crystal represents your intuitive center, the gateway to your inner wisdom and heightened perception. You notice that the crystal is pulsating with energy, symbolizing the potential for expanding your consciousness and connecting with your innate intuition.

You reach out and touch the crystal, feeling a surge of insight and awareness. With this connection, you realize that you have the power to open up your intuitive center, allowing you to cultivate a deeper understanding of yourself and the world around you.

Direct Suggestions

As you continue to relax, know that you have the ability to open up your intuitive center and enhance your perception beyond the physical senses. Each day, you are becoming more and more skilled at recognizing and trusting your intuition, allowing you to navigate your life with greater clarity and wisdom.

Indirect Suggestions

It's fascinating how the mind can develop new strategies for expanding consciousness, such as engaging in meditation, mindfulness practices, or exploring various forms of spiritual and personal growth.

Embedded Commands

Trust in your inner strength and ability to open up your intuitive center and enhance your perception. Allow your intuition to guide you toward opportunities and experiences that can help you cultivate a deeper understanding of yourself and the world around you.

Post Hypnotic Suggestions

From this moment forward, whenever you need to remind yourself of your ability to open up your intuitive center, simply take a moment to pause and recall the image of the magnificent crystal that symbolizes your inner wisdom and heightened perception. You have the tools and resources necessary to effectively expand your consciousness and connect with your innate intuition.

Awakener

Now, it's time to return to full awareness. I will count from one to five, and with each number, you will become more and more awake, bringing with you the positive suggestions and feelings of relaxation.

1 - Beginning to awaken, feeling rejuvenated.
2 - Becoming more alert and aware.
3 - Feeling your body and mind re-energize.
4 - Almost completely awake, feeling refreshed and revitalized.
5 - Fully awake and alert, ready to face the day with a renewed sense of insight and awareness.

Take a moment to stretch and enjoy the feeling of relaxation and rejuvenation. Remember, you possess the power to open up your intuitive center, empowering you to live a fulfilling and insightful life.

THIRD EYE 2

Pre-talk

Welcome to this hypnotic journey designed to guide you toward awakening your inner sense of intuition and expanding your awareness beyond the physical realm. Before we begin, please ensure that you are in a comfortable and safe environment, free from any distractions. Make sure you are seated or lying down in a relaxed position. Remember, hypnosis is a natural state of relaxation and focus, and you are always in control. This session is about guiding you to discover your own inner resources for enhancing your consciousness and connecting with your innate intuitive abilities.

Induction

As you begin to settle into a comfortable position, allow your eyes to gently close and take a few deep breaths. Inhale through your nose, and exhale through your mouth. With each breath, feel your body becoming more and more relaxed. Allow any tension or stress to simply melt away as you focus on your breathing.

As you continue to breathe, imagine a calming, protective light surrounding your entire body. This light represents a sense of inner wisdom and tranquility. As the light envelops you, feel the muscles in your body relax, and allow this calming, protective light to release any tension that may be stored.

Deepener

The soothing light continues to move through your body, from your head down to your toes. With each breath, this calming, protective light is filling your body, leaving you completely relaxed and at ease.

Now, imagine yourself walking along a serene, mystical forest path. The vibrant colors of the trees and the gentle sounds of the forest create a sense of peace and wonder. As you explore the forest, you feel more and more relaxed, fully embracing this magical environment.

Metaphors

As you continue to walk through the forest, you come across a tranquil pond, reflecting the light of the moon. This pond represents your inner sense of intuition, the gateway to your inner wisdom and expanded awareness. You notice that the water in the pond is shimmering with a soft, radiant light, symbolizing the potential for awakening your consciousness and connecting with your innate intuitive abilities.

You kneel down and touch the water, feeling a surge of insight and clarity. With this connection, you realize that you have the power to awaken your inner sense of intuition, allowing you to cultivate a deeper understanding of yourself and the world around you.

Direct Suggestions

As you continue to relax, know that you have the ability to awaken your inner sense of intuition and expand your awareness beyond the physical realm. Each day, you are becoming more and more skilled at recognizing and trusting your intuition, allowing you to navigate your life with greater clarity and wisdom.

Indirect Suggestions

You might find it intriguing how the mind can develop new strategies for enhancing consciousness, such as engaging in meditation, mindfulness practices, or exploring various forms of spiritual and personal growth.

Embedded Commands

Believe in your inner strength and ability to awaken your inner sense of intuition and expand your awareness. Allow your intuition to guide you toward opportunities and experiences that can help you cultivate a deeper understanding of yourself and the world around you.

Post Hypnotic Suggestions

From this moment forward, whenever you need to remind yourself of your ability to awaken your inner sense of intuition, simply take a moment to pause and recall the image of the tranquil pond that symbolizes your inner wisdom and expanded awareness. You have the tools and resources necessary to effectively enhance your consciousness and connect with your innate intuitive abilities.

Awakener

Now, it's time to return to full awareness. I will count from one to five, and with each number, you will become more and more awake, bringing with you the positive suggestions and feelings of relaxation.

1 - Beginning to awaken, feeling rejuvenated.
2 - Becoming more alert and aware.
3 - Feeling your body and mind re-energize.
4 - Almost completely awake, feeling refreshed and revitalized.
5 - Fully awake and alert, ready to face the day with a renewed sense of insight and awareness.

Take a moment to stretch and enjoy the feeling of relaxation and rejuvenation. Remember, you possess the power to awaken your inner sense of intuition, empowering you to live a fulfilling and insightful life.

RELAXATION 1

Pre-talk

Welcome to this hypnotic journey designed to guide you toward a deep state of relaxation and inner peace. Before we begin, please ensure that you are in a comfortable and safe environment, free from any distractions. Make sure you are seated or lying down in a relaxed position. Remember, hypnosis is a natural state of relaxation and focus, and you are always in control. This session is about guiding you to discover your own inner resources for achieving relaxation and cultivating a sense of calm in your daily life.

Induction

As you begin to settle into a comfortable position, allow your eyes to gently close and take a few deep breaths. Inhale through your nose, and exhale through your mouth. With each breath, feel your body becoming more and more relaxed. Allow any tension or stress to simply melt away as you focus on your breathing.

As you continue to breathe, imagine a soothing, warm light surrounding your entire body. This light represents a sense of calm and tranquility. As the light envelops you, feel the muscles in your body relax, and allow this soothing, warm light to release any tension that may be stored.

Deepener

The calming light continues to move through your body, from your head down to your toes. With each breath, this soothing, warm light is filling your body, leaving you completely relaxed and at ease.

Now, imagine yourself in a serene, peaceful garden. The vibrant colors of the flowers and the gentle sound of a nearby stream create a sense of tranquility and wonder. As you explore the garden, you feel more and more relaxed, fully embracing this soothing environment.

Metaphors

As you continue to walk through the garden, you come across a comfortable bench, inviting you to sit down and rest. This bench represents the place within you where you can always find relaxation and inner peace. You sit down on the bench, feeling a sense of calm and serenity wash over you, symbolizing your ability to achieve relaxation whenever you need it.

Direct Suggestions

As you continue to relax, know that you have the ability to find relaxation and inner peace in your daily life. Each day, you are becoming more and more skilled at recognizing the moments when you need to pause and allow yourself to relax, enabling you to cultivate a sense of calm and balance.

Indirect Suggestions

It's interesting how the mind can develop new strategies for achieving relaxation, such as engaging in mindfulness practices, deep breathing exercises, or simply taking a moment to pause and appreciate the beauty around you.

Embedded Commands

Trust in your inner strength and ability to find relaxation and inner peace whenever you need it. Allow yourself to embrace the moments of stillness and tranquility, nurturing a sense of balance and harmony in your life.

Post Hypnotic Suggestions

From this moment forward, whenever you need to remind yourself of your ability to relax, simply take a moment to pause and touch your thumb and index finger together. This simple gesture will serve as an anchor, helping you recall the feelings of relaxation and serenity you experienced while sitting on the bench in the peaceful garden. You have the tools and resources necessary to effectively achieve relaxation and cultivate a sense of calm in your daily life.

Awakener

Now, it's time to return to full awareness. I will count from one to five, and with each number, you will become more and more awake, bringing with you the positive suggestions and feelings of relaxation.

1 - Beginning to awaken, feeling rejuvenated.
2 - Becoming more alert and aware.
3 - Feeling your body and mind re-energize.
4 - Almost completely awake, feeling refreshed and revitalized.
5 - Fully awake and alert, ready to face the day with a renewed sense of calm and balance.

Take a moment to stretch and enjoy the feeling of relaxation and rejuvenation. Remember, you possess the power to find relaxation and inner peace whenever you need it, empowering you to live a fulfilling and balanced life.

RELAXATION 2

Pre-talk

Welcome to this hypnotic journey designed to guide you toward achieving a deep state of relaxation and inner calm. Before we begin, please ensure that you are in a comfortable and safe environment, free from any distractions. Make sure you are seated or lying down in a relaxed position. Remember, hypnosis is a natural state of relaxation and focus, and you are always in control. This session is about guiding you to discover your own inner resources for cultivating relaxation and serenity in your daily life.

Induction

As you begin to settle into a comfortable position, allow your eyes to gently close and take a few deep breaths. Inhale through your nose, and exhale through your mouth. With each breath, feel your body becoming more and more relaxed. Allow any tension or stress to simply melt away as you focus on your breathing.

As you continue to breathe, imagine a comforting, gentle breeze surrounding your entire body. This breeze represents a sense of calm and tranquility. As the breeze envelops you, feel the muscles in your body relax, and allow this comforting, gentle breeze to release any tension that may be stored.

Deepener

The soothing breeze continues to move through your body, from your head down to your toes. With each breath, this comforting, gentle breeze is filling your body, leaving you completely relaxed and at ease.

Now, imagine yourself on a beautiful, secluded beach. The sound of the waves and the warmth of the sun create a sense of peace and serenity. As you explore the beach, you feel more and more relaxed, fully embracing this soothing environment.

Metaphors

As you continue to walk along the beach, you come across a cozy hammock, gently swaying between two palm trees. This hammock represents the place within you where you can always find relaxation and inner calm. You lie down in the hammock, feeling a sense of peace and serenity wash over you, symbolizing your ability to achieve relaxation whenever you need it.

Direct Suggestions

As you continue to relax, know that you have the ability to find relaxation and inner calm in your daily life. Each day, you are becoming more and more skilled at recognizing the moments when you need to pause and allow yourself to relax, enabling you to cultivate a sense of balance and serenity.

Indirect Suggestions

It's fascinating how the mind can develop new strategies for achieving relaxation, such as engaging in mindfulness practices, deep breathing exercises, or simply taking a moment to pause and appreciate the beauty around you.

Embedded Commands

Believe in your inner strength and ability to find relaxation and inner calm whenever you need it. Allow yourself to embrace the moments of stillness and tranquility, nurturing a sense of balance and harmony in your life.

Post Hypnotic Suggestions

From this moment forward, whenever you need to remind yourself of your ability to relax, simply take a moment to pause and gently press your palm against your heart. This simple gesture will serve as an anchor, helping you recall the feelings of relaxation and serenity you experienced while lying in the hammock on the peaceful beach. You have the tools and resources necessary to effectively achieve relaxation and cultivate a sense of calm in your daily life.

Awakener

Now, it's time to return to full awareness. I will count from one to five, and with each number, you will become more and more awake, bringing with you the positive suggestions and feelings of relaxation.

1 - Beginning to awaken, feeling rejuvenated.
2 - Becoming more alert and aware.
3 - Feeling your body and mind re-energize.
4 - Almost completely awake, feeling refreshed and revitalized.
5 - Fully awake and alert, ready to face the day with a renewed sense of calm and balance.

Take a moment to stretch and enjoy the feeling of relaxation and rejuvenation. Remember, you possess the power to find relaxation and inner calm whenever you need it, empowering you to live a fulfilling and balanced life.

ABOUT THE AUTHOR

Joseph E. (Joey) Sapp, JD CCH-AP, is the CEO of LEGAL WRITING USA. Since 1992, Joey has been involved in well over 100 trials ranging from sexual assault to police/official misconduct. He retired from active private trial practice undefeated in jury trials as sole counsel.

In 1998, he was co-counsel for the defendant Billy Crowder in what has been dubbed the 'Tomato Patch Murder.' Court TV, as well as other media outlets broadcast documentaries on this infamous trial; multiple books have been written on it.

He is a co-founder of Hope House Recovery, Inc., a private halfway house/recovery residence for men in Athens, Georgia. Along with fellow co-founder Matt Minshew, he designed an award winning program which was certified by the State of Georgia. The Hope House has been in continuous operation since 1998.

In 2015, he served as a founding executive member of the Ubuntu Party USA, the American arm of the Ubuntu Party International, a trans-national political party holding elective office in multiple countries.

In 2019, Joey became the director of a 60+ bed rehabilitation facility operated by the largest provider of halfway house/transition services in the United States where he supervised and counseled addicts and alcoholics in transition on issues of employment, independent living, legal issues, and recovery.

He has been, and continues to be, responsible for removing corrupt officials from office and other positions of authority, and he provides litigation support to litigants, attorneys and law firms nationwide.

He is the author of numerous books to include: "How to Avoid Arrest" - "The Principles Behind the Steps" - "Thirty Days of Hope" - "Hypnosis & the Law" & "Navigating the Perils of Pseudolaw in America".

EDUCATION

1990, Associates in Computer Science and Electronic Engineering equivalency US Army Signal School as a 39E.

1996, Bachelor of Science in Political Science with concentrations in Judicial Process and Public Policy from Georgia Southern University.

2000, Juris Doctor with concentrations in Public Policy and the Law of Legislative Government from the University of Georgia School of Law.

2020, Clinical Hypnotist Certification from KEW Academy.

2021, Certified Clinical Hypnotherapist from Transform Destiny.

2023, Advanced Hypnosis Practitioner certification by the International Certification Board of Clinical Hypnotists.

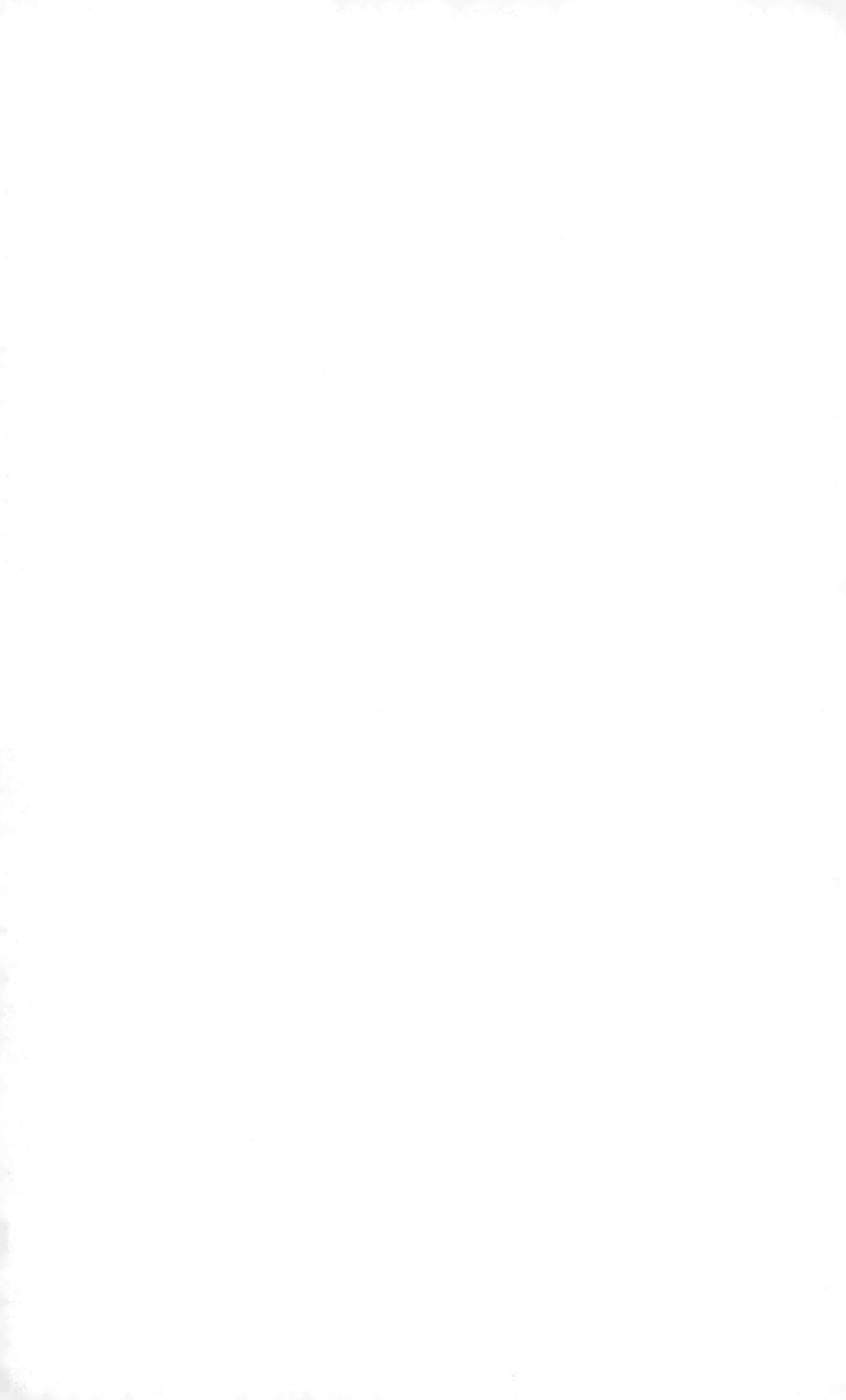

Printed in the USA
CPSIA information can be obtained
at www.ICGtesting.com
LVHW011604030624
782149LV00009B/382